# Exclusively Mother's Milk

A sure guide for breastfeeding working mothers

Martha Raymond

# HOW TO USE THIS BOOK

This book is packed with loads of information compiled from one on one interviews with nursing mothers, nurses, lactation experts. Their various experiences and recommendation have been put together in this book to help mothers alike.

This book have been put together to help mothers know what to do to prepare for transitioning from breastfeeding at home to trying to do so while working, despite the fact that many women who join the workforce within the first few months after the birth of their children make the combination of breastfeeding and working their goal.

# EXCLUSIVE BREASTFEEDING

Jennifer gave birth to her first child at the age of 26, like most first time mothers she lacked the experience of exclusively breastfeeding her child for 6 months. During this period she pursued a nursing degree while spending less time with her son. Three years later Jennifer decides to make up by exclusively breastfeeding her second son. When interviewed on her desire to make this change she said "I make this decision not because I suddenly have all the time in the world but I am more motivated because I am more aware of the benefits and I constantly see the impact this decision has on my son. One of the benefits I have come to understand is that my son easily puts on weight and does not experience nausea and diarrhea as compared to my first son who I fed using baby formulas".

The World Health Organization (WHO) advises breastfeeding exclusively for the first six months, then continuing with supplemental foods until the child is two years old or older. To guarantee that children grow, develop, and reach their full potential, they must have adequate nutrition from infancy and the early years of childhood. Since breast milk is the finest source of nutrition for a baby, it is well-acknowledged that breastfeeding is good for both the mother and baby.

Exclusive breastfeeding, with the exception of vitamins, minerals, and medications, is the practice of giving infants only breast milk during the first six months of life. No other liquids, food, tea, or herbal remedies are given to the infants during this time. One of the best strategies to ensure the well-being and survival of a child is to breastfeed. Less than half of infants under 6 months are exclusively breastfed. The best nourishment for babies is breast milk. Antibodies found in it aid in preventing a number of prevalent pediatric ailments, and it is secure and hygienic.

# BREAST MILK

The human mammary glands generate breast milk, a complex fluid. It has a well-balanced combination of nutrients, immune cells, antibodies, enzymes, and hormones. As the baby grows, the composition alters to accommodate their changing dietary requirements. Colostrum, the first milk produced after delivery, is a source of immune-boosting antibodies and proteins that also aid in establishing the gut micro biota of the new-born. The milk changes to contain more fat and energy as the infant gets older. Breast milk's unique nutrients boost the infant's growth, cognitive development, and immune system, providing a host of health advantages.

## Types of Breast Milk

As a baby develops, a mother primarily produces one of three types of breast milk:

**Colostrum:** During the first several days following childbirth, this is the first milk produced. It is thick and yellowish in color, and it is full with nutrients, proteins, and antibodies that assist the infant be protected and develop their immune system.

**Transitional Milk:** The content and abundance of colostrum change as it transitions. It is known as transitional milk and has rising percentages of fat, lactose, and calories. The baby's digestive tract is assisted by this milk in adjusting to more complex foods.

**Mature Milk:** Approximately two weeks later, mature milk starts to be produced. Although it contains a larger fat content, it is thinner than colostrum and transitional milk. Foremilk, a watery component of mature milk, and both mature milk and hind milk, which is higher in fat and provide nutrients and energy, relieve thirst.

Each of these varieties of breast milk is essential for supplying the infant's varying dietary and developmental demands.

## Benefits of breast milk for the baby

Your infant receives a healthy start in life from breast milk. For around the first six months, it is the only nourishment your infant requires.

- Breast milk is always pure, uncontaminated, and at the proper temperature.
- In order to meet your baby's evolving needs, your breast milk will vary over time.
- Your baby's immune system is strengthened by breast milk.
- Your kid gets more from breastfeeding than just nourishment.
- Your baby can feel, smell, and see you when you are nursing him or her nearby.
- This aids in the development of a strong, loving link between you and your child.

## Helps Prevent Postpartum Depression

With the assistance of the prolactin hormones, breastfeeding lowers blood pressure, improves sleep quality, reduces anxiety in moms, and lowers negative mood. These effects all work to lessen the chance of postpartum depression in mothers.

## Immunity

Antibodies from the mother's breast milk are often passed on to the new born. These antibodies aid in the development of a robust immune system, reducing the risk of the infant contracting infections like gastroenteritis and ear infections as well as illnesses common in children including obesity, asthma, and pneumonia.

## Psychological Growth

A baby's intellect seems to develop better when they are exclusively breastfed. This is because breast milk naturally supplies the essential elements needed by the baby.

## Affordability and Availability

Breast milk is generally affordable. It doesn't need to be purchased because it is produced directly from the mother and fed through the mother's breast. It is generally available. This is because breast milk doesn't have a specific time it is being produced; instead it is produced at all time making breast milk available at all times.

# Benefits for the Mother

## Natural means of family planning

Breastfeeding acts as a natural technique of family planning that aids in spacing out children. The lactation amenorrhea method is what it is known as. Because the hormone prolactin, which is responsible for the production of breast milk, is secreted more frequently when a mother breastfeeds her child exclusively, this method of family planning is effective in preventing pregnancy and menstruation in these women.

## Enables Bonding

The body produces prolactin and oxytocin when a mother breastfeeds her infant. A calm, maternal sensation brought on by oxytocin enables moms to unwind and concentrate on their children. It strengthens your bond with your infant and fosters a deep sense of love and affection between you two.

## Economic benefits

The total price of household food bills is decreased by avoiding the need to purchase infant milk formulae thanks to exclusive breastfeeding.

It also assists in lowering healthcare expenses. In this situation, unlike breast milk, which is natural, certain babies could be allergic to particular components used in creating milk formulas, resulting in increased expense.

# BREASTFEEDING WITHOUT NURSING

Emily a mother of three is accustomed to the midnight feeding practice. She has rocked and cuddled one of her three kids back to sleep for more than ten years in a dimly lit nursery. With her youngest, though, Emily hears the whirr of a breast pump removing her breast milk as the infant in her arms drinks from a bottle rather than the cooing and sucking of a nursing baby.

One of many new parents, Emily pumps her breast milk solely rather than nursing her child directly. She says, "The first three weeks of nursing were hell." Due to her inverted nipples, her kid was having difficulty latching and wasn't eating well. She disliked the idea of having to take formula supplements, which was what her doctor had advised.

She explains, "I did not want to supplement and I really wanted to give her breast milk exclusively for as long as I could." However, because her infant was not gaining weight, she made the decision to begin pumping in order to gauge the precise amount of milk that her child was consuming.

Despite being quite disappointed, she later realized that exclusively pumping was the best course of action for her. But not everyone can nurse naturally; for a variety of reasons, many people find it uncomfortable, painful, or even impossible.

Emily was able to breastfeed and did so for her two previous children until her job and other obstacles got in the way, but breastfeeding this time around didn't work and also didn't fit into her hectic schedule.

## Exclusive Pumping

Exclusive pumping refers to a feeding technique when breast milk is only obtained for bottle feeding by utilizing a breast pump (or hand expression). Moms may opt to exclusively breastfeed for a variety of reasons. Medical necessity or personal inclinations are two possible explanations. For some, it's the best of all worlds: Baby receives the advantages of breast milk, and Mom has the freedom to bottle-feed (and share that burden with others!). However, exclusive pumping is not always a quick or easy fix.

## Pumping and Not Breastfeeding: The Challenges

Though only pumping may seem like a better solution, it has a number of drawbacks, such as:

- Time to pump
- After pumping, you must use a bottle to feed your baby
- Cleaning bottle and pump parts
- How much a breast pump, bottles, and supplies will cost
- When traveling, finding a place to pump

## The Advantages of Breastfeeding vs. Pumping

Emily quickly understood how much preparation and thought went into simply pumping instead of breastfeeding. You do need to follow a fairly strict schedule when pumping. When you need to pump, you need to schedule everything around that time, Emily advises. She always has a manual pump and a nipple shield in her baby's diaper bag in case of emergencies, just in case she needs to nurse.

However, for Emily, the additional work is worthwhile. Parents generally concur that there are more advantages to pumping than disadvantages. These advantages consist of:

- Independence to travel
- Ability to observe how much milk a baby consumes Flexibility in enabling others to feed the infant consumes.
- Freedom and adaptability

Some women may discover that, despite direct nursing, they sometimes require a pump in order to boost their milk supply. If parents exclusively breastfeed, adding pumping to the routine also enables them to be away from their infants at a typical mealtime and still make milk for later.

The absence of direct breast contact with the infant is the main distinction between mothers who both nurse and pump and those who solely pump. Myers was concerned about this since it meant she wouldn't have the same emotional connection with her child as she had with her older children while nursing them.

But she adds, "I observed despite I was not nursing but bottle feeding my baby I still was able to spend time bonding with my baby". She enjoyed being able to monitor her baby's exact calorie intake as well. She claims that "this really removed the guesswork. It helped me know how much food my baby needed to be full. This is a huge comfort for moms who worry that their kid isn't eating enough because they don't make enough milk".

Based on observation, infants who are bottle-fed often consume more milk than those who are nursed; exclusively breastfed infants within the ages of one month and six months consume an average of 25oz (750 mL) per day, while a typical range of breast milk contains between 1 and 3oz.

Daily bottle intake ranges from 19 to 30 ounces (570 to 900 mL).Though each infant will have a different amount of breast or bottle feeding. Overfeeding is more likely due to the bottle's quick, reliable milk flow.

# BREAST PUMP

Nicole a female nurse who juggles between her job and caring for her daughter says "with my first child, I made the error of underestimating the value of my breast pump. When it came to choosing a breast pump, I was, like many other mothers, dazed and confused. There are so many options: manual, electric, single, double, and hospital-grade, the list is endless. When you've never done it before, it can be difficult to determine what you need".

According to her, during prenatal classes, questions about breast pumps are frequently the most common. She was asked to respond to a few of the most typical queries women have when shopping for and utilizing breast pumps, based on her experience. Some of the questions include:

## Can I Use A Breast Pump With My Health Insurance?

Yes! Healthcare insurers must provide coverage for breast pumps under the Affordable Care Act. Not all expectant mothers are aware of this because it is still relatively new. Speak to your health insurance provider about the coverage options since each plan is unique. Inquire about the following things:

- Which breast pumps are covered, and what types and brands?
- Should I ask my doctor for a prescription?
- Before my baby is born, can I purchase the pump through my insurance provider?
- Do I need to speak with a particular durable medical equipment (DME) provider (such as a pharmacy or medical supply company) in order to get a breast pump paid for by my insurance?

For a good, basic double electric pump, the majority of insurance providers will pay. A little fee can be required if you want an improved model or a rental pump with several users. Comparable situations include prescription drug coverage for generic versus name-brand medications.

## Which Breast Pump Is The Best For Me?

To begin with, a breast pump is not strictly necessary. Thousands of years without pumps, women have nursed. Because of this, it's okay if you choose not to use one. You should probably think about an electric pump if you work outside the home to save time. Whether you select a single or double depends on how comfortable you feel.

Consider how you'll employ your breast pump.
The pump should be suitable for the application. A manual pump may be sufficient if you only want to breastfeed once or twice per week and will be at home with the baby for several weeks or months. Don't write off manual pumps because there are some excellent ones out there

I advise renting a hospital-grade pump if your baby needs to spend time in the Neonatal Intensive Care Unit (NICU) because you'll probably need to pump eight or more times each day to provide milk for your infant. Although you can convert to a personal pump later, you'll benefit from the extra power a larger an electric pump provides while you're still building up your milk supply.

Most women only require a hospital-grade pump during their time in the NICU or if they have low milk supply in the past. They can be cumbersome and heavy to transport!

The plastic pieces you place over your breasts are called flanges, and they are not universally applicable. For milk expression, the pump draws the nipple into the flange. The flanges must fit snugly to prevent pain and abrasions that could cause an infection. The majority of women will, but not all, fit the standard-size flange. Both in-store and through direct contact with the business, you may purchase them in various sizes. A different size might be necessary if you start pumping and find it uncomfortable.

## Must I clean my breast pump after each use?

For the health of both you and your baby, properly washing your breast pump is essential. But whether you're working or traveling, it might be challenging. The advice we give women most frequently is to store the pump kit in the refrigerator with the milk if there is room for it at work. You won't need to wash it after every usage if you do it that way, best to wash it at home during the night hours. You'll get a lot of time back during the workday by doing this.

Your pump kit doesn't require any special cleaning products. Water and soap will both do the trick. Even the dishwasher will work with it. It would be ideal if your dishwasher had a sanitized cycle. In order to disinfect your pump, you can also purchase microwaveable bags. Many of these bags have a limit on how many times they can be used. Ensure that you adhere to the directions.

Invest on items made for storing breast milk rather than formula when purchasing things. When you freeze and thaw the milk, some formula storage bags' seams may not hold the milk together as well. After spilling breast milk, you will never again cry over spilt milk. Breast milk can be expressed manually or mechanically. Breast pumps come in a variety of styles and are available for purchase or rental. The one you pick will depend on how you want to utilize it.

# Why you might require a breast pump?

If your child is sick or preterm, for instance, or if you have to return to work, you might need to express milk when you are away from them. Additionally, you might express milk if your breasts feel uncomfortable full or to combine with your baby's first solid foods. Many women express milk and keep it in the freezer for emergency situations.

Some women simply need to express themselves for a short while, while others intend to do so permanently. For various levels of usage, there are many breast pumps.

As soon as you are able, you should begin pumping if your baby cannot be breastfed from birth (for instance, because they are premature or have specific needs). If you have many children, ask your pediatrician or lactation consultant about using a breast pump to increase your supply. You can begin pumping early and freeze the milk if you want to return to the workforce.

# Breast Pumps' Various Types

An over-the-nipple suction cup, a funnel, and a collection bottle make up a breast pump. To encourage your milk to start flowing, the pump imitates your baby's sucking motion. It collects the milk in the bottle once it has been extracted.

Breast pumps come in three main varieties:
1. **Manual:** To withdraw the milk, squeeze a handle repeatedly.
2. **Electric:** The device pumps on its own.
   - **Single electric:** This type of pump only pumps one breast at a time and is powered by a motor that may be electric or battery-operated.
   - **Double electric:** These can simultaneously pump both breasts and are powered by a motor, which reduces the amount of time it takes to pump.
3. **Hospital grade:** A barrier separates the milk collection kit from the pump mechanism, keeping the milk away from the air and any potential germs. Several women might share this "closed system" pump.

Less than once a day or for a brief period of time, manual pumps is suitable for use. Furthermore, they are more covert. It could be beneficial to think about purchasing or hiring an electric breast pump if you intend to use the pump more frequently or for a longer period of time. Electric pumps allow you to simultaneously pump both breasts and operate more quickly and efficiently. With their second child, many women switch from a manual to an electric breast pump. Whatever you choose, make sure to get the best pump you can manage.

Different sized breast shields for breast pumps are available. A shield that is the proper size for you should be chosen. The sides will be scraped by the nipple if it is too small. If it's too large, the milk flow will be hampered and the areola will get uncomfortable from being dragged into the funnel. If you can easily and comfortably pump with your nipple inserted into the funnel, the shield is the proper size.

When putting your breast pump together and cleaning it, always follow the directions provided by the manufacturer. Immediately following usage, all breast pumps must be sterilized. Where to get a breast pump a breast pump can be rented or purchased. Even if you employ one, you must still purchase your own milk collection kit (the components of the pump that come into touch with the milk, such as the breast shield and collecting bottle), in order to prevent infection. The use of a used breast pump is not advised. Other methods of expressing milk, it is additionally possible to mix hand expressing and pumping to express milk. Your milk production may rise as a result.

## Pumping and milk storage

There are a few crucial stages to correctly pumping and storing breast milk:

1. Cleanliness: Make sure your pumping equipment is clean and sanitized, and wash your hands thoroughly before expressing milk.
2. Adhere to the instructions provided by the manufacturer when assembling and using the pump. Find a spot that is calm and relaxing where you can pump, ideally simulating your baby's feeding schedule.

3. Maintaining a healthy diet and staying hydrated will help your body produce more milk.

4. Utilize food-grade, BPA-free storage containers. Breast milk storage bags and glass or plastic containers with tight-fitting lids are both options.

5. Labeling: Indicate the expression date on each container. First in, first out means to use the oldest milk first.

6. Cooling: If you won't be using the milk right away, put it in the fridge or a cooler as soon as you can. Freshly pumped milk can be kept in the refrigerator for up to 4–8 days at a temperature of about 32–39°F (0–4°C).

7. Freezing: Within 24 hours, move milk to the freezer for extended preservation. At 0°F (-18°C) or colder, frozen milk can be kept for six to twelve months.

8. In the refrigerator overnight or under cool running water, you can thaw frozen milk. Never use a microwave since it may result in uneven heating and degrade crucial nutrients.
9. Gently stir the frozen milk to incorporate any cream that may have separated. Avoid shaking erratically.
10. Warming: Heat milk that has been refrigerated or thawed by submerging the container in warm water.

## Three methods for thawing breast milk

Nothing is more frustrating than freezing a bag of breast milk only to have the bag leak. Seeing your milk go to waste may be messy in addition to being painful. Here are three defrosting techniques for breast milk, along with tips on how to accomplish each one without losing any milk.

Frozen breast milk can be defrosted in one of three ways:

- Inside the fridge
- In cool water
- In a warm water

## In The Refrigerator

Best for Bottle preparation and later usage, Breast milk is best defrosted inside a refrigerator. However, it takes the longest for your milk to thaw in this manner. The amount of milk in the breast milk bag, the refrigerator's temperature, and the amount of other food present all affect how long it will take for the food to defrost. In general, take it out of the freezer and put it in the refrigerator for 12 to 24 hours before you need it defrosted.

To accomplish this, place your breast milk storage bag in a spick-and-span bowl and place it in the refrigerator to thaw. If you'd like, you can wrap it in plastic wrap in case of leaks to keep bacteria from getting into the breast milk. Once the milk has finished thawing you can now proceed with pouring it into a bottle. You might wish to utilize your breast shield as a funnel to reduce spills. After milk has finished thawing in the refrigerator, it should be used within 24 hours.

**Using Cold Water to Defrost Frozen Milk**

**Best for**: Not using all of the milk right now, but some of it. You can thaw milk in cold water if you aren't going to use all of the milk that is in the bag right away or if you are making bottles that will be consumed later and don't want to wait for it to defrost in the refrigerator.

Use this approach just for milk that you intend to consume within the following 24 hours. To thaw breast milk in cold water, follow these simple steps:

1. Prepare the water. When defrosting the milk, if a sink is nearby, run the water until it is cold, plug it, and then fill it with water to cover the surface.
2. Put the bag of breast milk into a fresh zip-top plastic bag if you're worried about leaks.

3. Any leaks will be caught by the zip-top bag, keeping the milk from being wasted. Thawing frozen breast milk in a silicone reusable breastfeeding bag is an additional option (because these bags don't leak).
4. Place the bag in the water, and then give it some time to sit there.
5. Remove the bag from the sink once it has thawed and pour the liquid into a bottle.
6. You ought to be able to detect if the breast milk bag leaked into the zip-top bag at this stage.
7. Pour it into the bottle you'll be using to administer food if it doesn't spill. As you transfer, you can utilize it as a funnel to prevent spills.
8. If the breast milk bag did leak, retain it in the plastic bag, unzip it, and delicately pour the milk into the bottle while holding it in place to prevent the milk that seeped into the zip-top bag from spilling out.

9. After that, remove the breast milk bag from the plastic bag. Any milk that spilled into the zip-top bag should then be poured into the bottle.

10.    When the milk has thawed, you have two options: you may reheat it up and give the baby right away, or you can pour it into bottles to keep in the fridge. The milk should be consumed two hours after it has been warmed.

## Using Warm Water to Thaw Frozen Milk

The milk should be used up immediately. Breast milk that is frozen and that you intend to use right away can be quickly and easily defrosted by putting it in warm water, which will also warm the milk. (Water should be lukewarm rather than too hot.) Once the breast milk has been warmed, you should only use this procedure if you intend to use the entire bag of milk.

You can do this by simply placing a bag of breast milk in warm water at the bottom of your sink or a clean bowl, waiting a short while, and then repeating the process described above.

Keep in mind that, unlike silicone reusable breast milk bags, plastic storage bags for breast milk should always be thrown away.

# CREATING A BALANCE BETWEEN MOTHERHOOD AND CAREER

Cathy, an outpatient therapist, declares that she is committed to continuing to breastfeed and give her children pumped breast milk for as long as she can. "I consider it my goal to make sure their nutritional needs are met because I am the primary source of nutrition for my girls, which is why I pump," she explains. They should get the greatest since it's best for them. My family comes first!"

As a PhD student, Cathy is aware of the challenges faced by working mothers who are also nursing; she manages to balance both roles by planning her time and keeping to it. "I would strongly advise struggling mothers to seek support from friends and family and a lactation consultant," said the doctor. When Cathy feels overwhelmed her lactation expert, helps her stay motivated. "My family and I appreciate her help and support very much! Being a mother and attending to your child's demands can be difficult, so it's crucial to have support, Cathy said. It shouldn't be stressful to nurse or pump; it should be joyful, Keep at it; I promise, things get better. The bond is also irreplaceable.  Cathy attributes her ability to remain upbeat and on task when the routine gets challenging to her husband and her mother. They serve as my pillars. Without them, I don't know what I would do.

## How to Balance Breastfeeding as a Working Mothers

Breastfeeding doesn't necessarily have to stop when work is resumed. If there is a policy in place and a code of ethics at the company, it will be easier to keep juggle breastfeeding and work together.

The mother requires knowledge, self-assurance in her abilities and rights, as well as crucial elements like family, social, and workplace support, in order to be able to work without having to cease breastfeeding.

The advantages of breastfeeding are recognized on a personal and societal level, supporting improved health and saving time and money on all fronts. In addition to the support offered by medical professionals, the community is full of resources for breastfeeding information and practices, and there are support groups where mothers with experience may help new mothers overcome challenges and successfully breastfeed.

Depending on whether you choose to breastfeed or give your infant a bottle, breastfeeding your baby might take on numerous shapes. Even better, you can alternate the two approaches and practice mixed breastfeeding. While making baby bottles for the remainder of the day, breastfeed in the morning and evenings.

Combining a professional life with breastfeeding can be challenging. Contrary to popular opinion, many women decide to discontinue breastfeeding when they return to work, although this is not always required. There are various choices for those who choose to continue breastfeeding:

Either mom chooses to provide infant milk in bottles instead of breastfeeding throughout the day (but continue to do so in the morning, evening, and at night). Although it is the most sensible option, it is also the most difficult. Because the milk flows more naturally from the bottle, sometimes this makes the child who prefers it lose interest. The benefit for the mother is that she will experience fewer restrictions during the day.

Alternatively, a working mother can preserve enough milk to prepare bottles of breast milk for her child the next day. Drawing fluid might take time, especially if it needs to be done; therefore this suggests having spare time while working.

## Challenges of Juggling Work and Breastfeeding

- **Time management:** Career-driven mothers frequently struggle to balance their hectic work schedules and breastfeeding schedules, which causes stress and weariness.
- **Lack of Support:** It can be challenging for moms to locate convenient locations and times to pump breast milk or nurse due to

rigid work environments and unsupportive co-workers.

- **Feelings of guilt:** Juggling breastfeeding and professional goals can make moms feel guilty because they worry about not giving their children or their jobs their complete attention.

- **Prejudice and Discrimination:** Some employers or co-workers may still have a negative mind set toward nursing mothers, which can be stressful and have an influence on a mother's self-confidence.

- **Physical discomfort:** A mother's comfort and self-esteem may be harmed by navigating business clothes and breast pumping equipment.

# Triumphs of Juggling Work and Breastfeeding

- **Feelings of Fulfillment**: A mother's self-esteem is boosted when she successfully manages her breastfeeding goals with her job aims.

- **Bonding and Connection**: Breastfeeding gives women exceptional opportunities to connect and bond with their children, which can be beneficial for both parties' general well-being.

- **Personal Development:** Overcoming the difficulties of breastfeeding and a career fosters personal development, assisting moms in becoming more flexible and resilient people.

- **Inspiration for Others:** Working mothers who successfully juggle all facets of their lives serve as role models for other women experiencing comparable difficulties.

Some of these victories highlight the fortitude and tenacity of career-driven mothers who successfully negotiate the challenges of pursuing their professional goals while caring for their infants through breastfeeding.

# WEANING YOUR BABY AFTER EXCLUSIVE BREAST FEEDING

Congratulations if you made it up to this phase, most mothers usually heave a sigh of relief at the arrival of this stage.

Whether you choose to wean your child or your breastfeeding journey ends unexpectedly, this milestone might introduce you to some unique circumstances. When it's time to wean your child there are some things that you might go through physically and emotionally. Your emotional state may astound you. Even for individuals who are relieved to no longer need to breastfeed or pump,

No matter how, when, or for what reason you weaned, it's crucial to be ready for these mood changes and to know you're not alone. Contact your provider and ask for treatment if you have feelings that have been impacting your lifestyle or way of life for more than a few weeks or if you feel down or hopeless. Although the depression may go away once your hormones are back to usual, post-weaning depression has the potential to go very bad. You can manage your emotional health with the aid of a healthcare professional and regain your sense of self.

## When is the ideal time to begin weaning my child?

The process of weaning is when you stop giving your infant breast milk. Introduce complementary foods with your breast milk to your baby at the age of 6 months as the very first step toward weaning. Breast milk is gradually replaced by various nutritious foods and drinks during the weaning process.

According to Helen a nurse, "After 6 months of age, your baby begins to need higher levels of certain nutrients, such as iron, zinc, and vitamins B and D, that she can't get from your breast milk or her own reserves alone."

However, introducing solids will only first supplement your baby's milk intake and gradually replace it. For many months to come, breast milk will be her main source of nourishment.

93% of the calories consumed by a typical seven-month-old child come from milk. Milk may still provide the equivalent of half of her daily caloric needs even at eleven to sixteen months old.

Despite the fact that she has begun eating solids and regardless of her age, there is no healthier milk for her, claims Helen.

The length of time it takes to wean the infant can depend on how long the mother and the baby choose to wait, as Helen notes: "When to stop breastfeeding is up to you." Do not let what your friends or family members are doing or saying, or even what strangers are saying, pressure you. Everything is based on what you and your kid believes is best.

## Stopping Breastfeeding

It's recommended to wean your infant off breast milk gradually when you decide to do so. In addition to putting your health at danger for engorgement, blocked ducts, or mastitis, abruptly stopping breastfeeding would be difficult for your baby's immunological and digestive systems to adjust to. It might also be emotionally challenging for you both.

## Is It Necessary For Me To Stop Nursing?

Sometimes mothers incorrectly believe they must quit nursing when they don't. Breastfeeding can be a wonderful method to maintain closeness while going through a significant transition in both of your life if you're returning to work. Nursing sessions can continue to be a special moment for you and your baby at the beginning or end of the day as you pump milk to feed your baby while working. As an alternative, you could pump milk to bring or send home if you're planning to take a trip without your child.

## Weaning After Six-Month

At about six months old, your baby will begin eating solid meals, and as time goes on, you'll notice a natural decrease in the frequency of her breastfeeding sessions. She probably won't need as many feeds in a day after a year, in addition to meals and nutritious snacks. If you would like to reduce your breastfeeding any further, you should do it gradually.

There are several strategies to divert your child's attention from a shift in her feeding habits. Instead, some mothers give a drink and a snack that you can share to foster a sense of intimacy. Altering your regular schedule, playing a favorite game, are other options. While it may take some kids longer than others to adjust to the change, things will get better over time. Asking for advice from your healthcare provider is usually beneficial if you're having any issues weaning.

## Weaning Naturally

The weaning procedure will probably be prolonged and slow if you decide to allow your toddler to determine when to stop breastfeeding (often referred to as baby-led weaning or natural-term breastfeeding). She'll probably have fewer and shorter feeds as the months go by, and some mothers say their kids just lose interest after a while.

At the age of four, my daughter began to wean herself, recalls Sarah. By age three and a half, she started to feed much less frequently. Then, it appeared as though she had forgotten we were on vacation. Though she understands the milk disappears after six months, she still tries to latch on occasionally.

You ought to have enough time for your body to adjust, so you won't likely suffer any painful engorgement. However, you could find it emotionally challenging, so schedule lots of time for cuddling and bonding activities.

"Due to the fact that my baby was exclusively breastfed it was easier for him to be weaned naturally. I didn't want to abruptly stop him," says Kelly, a mother of one. He stopped being interested around age two. Despite the fact that I was pretty emotional, it was the ideal situation for us.

It's ideal to continue breastfeeding for as long as possible, but there are occasions when you must stop for health reasons or because you are unable to care for yourself and the baby simultaneously.

If you've been exclusively breastfeeding your baby up until this point, you'll almost probably need to pump out milk in order to prevent your breasts from getting uncomfortable and engorged. For this, some women find breast pumps to be the most convenient, while others prefer to perform the task by hand. Again, you should only express as much as is necessary to relieve any discomfort; you don't want to stimulate your body's ability to make more milk.

Your breasts may first feel sensitive and swollen, but they soon adjust. The feedback inhibitor of lactation (FIL) is a substance found in your breast milk. FIL instructs your body to reduce production when your baby stops nursing, but it could take just a few days or even weeks for your breasts to adapt.

www.ingramcontent.com/pod-product-compliance
Lightning Source LLC
Chambersburg PA
CBHW062300290526
45794CB00006B/2641